Put an End to Panic Attacks

An Amazing Analytical Account

Written by
Alec C Moir

ISBN: 9781724055118

Introduction

This is the third book I've written about panic attacks. Even though they are all more or less updates to the previous ones, with a lot more new content.

This delicate subject, still needs addressing because to date: September 2018, it still doesn't look like there's going to be any drastic change in the health industry anytime soon.

Apart from: Different medication that is, but that's defeating the object of what this book's about. Which is: Curing yourself from panic attacks, together with all the other temporarily related conditions associated with stress. Such as:

Depression
Anxiety
Aching joints
Fear of dying
Palpitations
Sweating
Hot flushes
Phobias
Trembling
Fear of being alone
Muscle Spasms
Vision Disorders
Numbness
Loss of concentration
Breathing Difficulties
House bound
Nervous Tension
Fear of loud noises
Brain fog

The list goes on and on, because that's how severe your: shall we say temporarily readjustments, really makes you feel.

That's why I called this book: "Put an End to Panic Attacks," because it really is a powerfully, simple, drug free and natural way of curing yourself from stress related symptoms full stop.

Chapter 1

You'll be pleased to know at this point that: You're well on your way to getting your life back to a normal functioning, give yourself a round of applause, for seeking out a natural alternative.

I would like to also reassure you that: You are not on your own. Panic attacks are one of many related symptoms, that fall into the same category… stress.

Millions of people are suffering from stress related symptoms everyday, and are going through the same sort of feelings you are having at this moment.

But the sad fact is: They will undoubtedly continue to suffer from panic attacks, until doctors start to realize that their advice coupled with sedatives and beta-blockers, just don't work for the long term effect.

Even though the doctors have probably told you that: the feelings you are having at the moment are completely natural. I am going to explain to you in detail, why you are having these symptoms in the first place.

How to avoid them in the future, and how you can easily cure yourself from panic attacks, and all the other stress related symptom once and for all.

The first few pages of this book, give you a brief encounter of the first panic attacks I started experiencing years ago, and went on suffering almost daily for two and half years.

My main reason for including my detailed experience, was for you to be able to relate to this short story, as more than likely all the symptoms will fit your's like a glove.

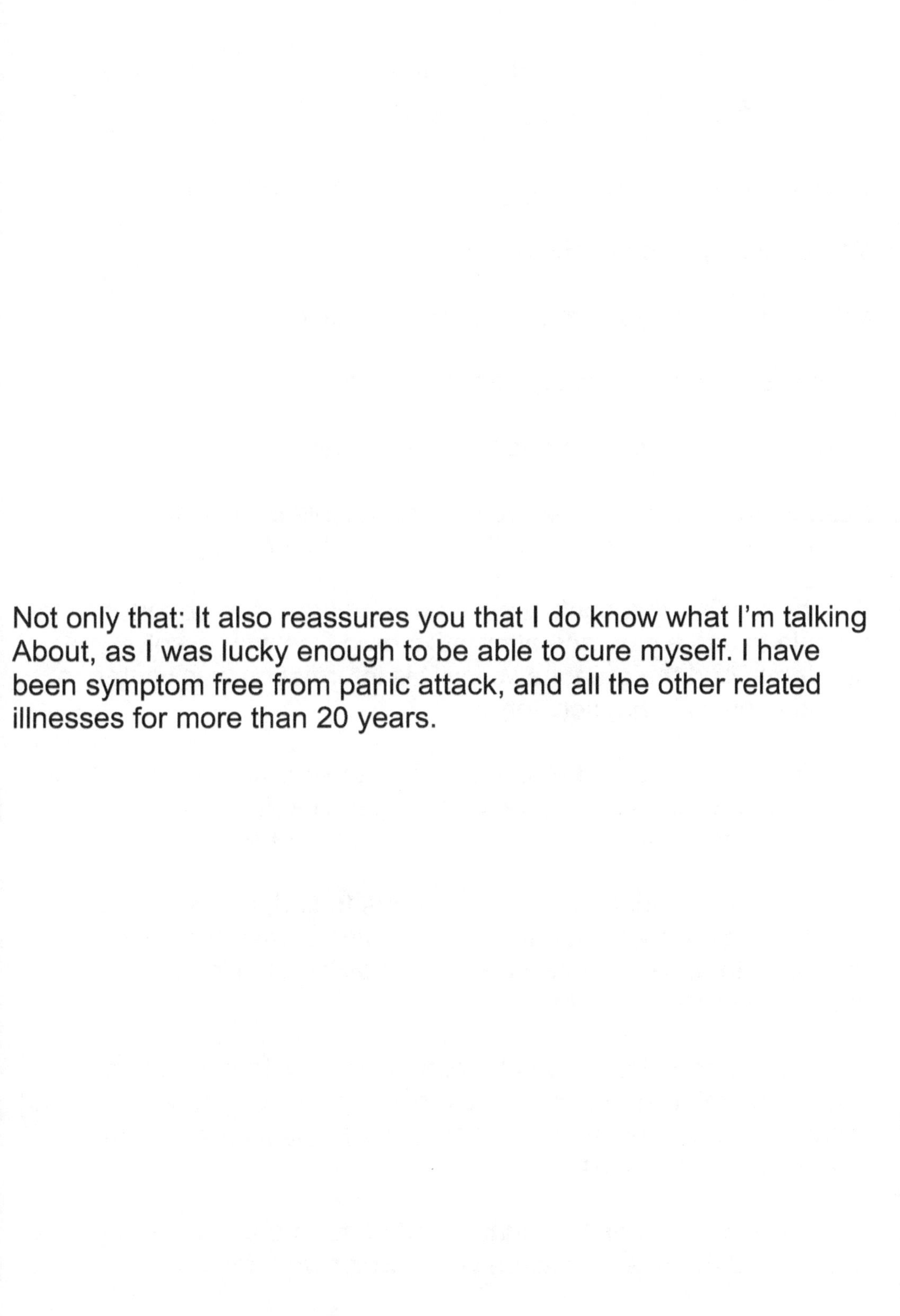

Not only that: It also reassures you that I do know what I'm talking About, as I was lucky enough to be able to cure myself. I have been symptom free from panic attack, and all the other related illnesses for more than 20 years.

Chapter 2
Some of the benefits you will learn

How you ended up with panic attacks in the first place?

What brings panic attacks on?

What is the best types of food to eat for panic attacks?

How to stop panic attacks dead in their tracks?

How to cure your panic attacks once and for all?

I can guarantee that once you start to put this information into practice: you will start to feel the benefits immediately.

Just by reading this book, you've given yourself the opportunity to be able to use a safe and alternative drug free way to solve your problems. And the great news is: This information was written to provide you with that solution.

This is your chance to be able to return to your normal way of life, to start enjoying yourself again, without having the thoughts of having a panic attacks lurking about over your head.

This information took me over two years to find, although I must say it was quite by accident. I was reading something entirely unrelated to panic attacks when it hit me like a brick. I realised then, my search was over.

I call this information a secret, because the doctors for some reason of their own, either don't know or won't tell you about it, and I must admit, I've never read about it in any publication about stress related illnesses.

All I do know for definite is that it worked for me and I'm living proof of that, and there is no reason why it won't work for you.

Chapter 3
A Step in The Right Direction

You'll be surprised to know: Panic attacks and all the other stress related symptoms, are mainly due to you having a chemical imbalance in your body. which could and does happen to tens of thousands of people on a daily basis.

Most of the time this will go unnoticed, or the person might feel a bit under the weather for a few weeks, until the chemicals have a chance to get back to their normal way of functioning.

You've more than likely heard the old saying, a hundred times before, by people you meet on the street, or by friends and relatives, "I don't know what's the matter with me just lately, I must be going through the change."

More often than not: they probably are going through some form of chemical change, depending on their circumstances. If you have allowed your body to receive a couple of hard knocks and not allowed it to function correctly.

This could be due to worrying too much about something, such as: work, bills, loved ones etc. Or you have started to eat irregularly, for example: Missed a few meals regularly.

Another example is: You might have gone on a strict diet, had a drastic change in your eating habits, started drinking a lot of liquids or even cut out saturated fats from your diet.

Some people like to socialise on a regular basis: Drinking alcohol regularly is often associated with panic attacks. But you'll be shocked when I reveal the culprit, alcohol is the innocent party in this case.

I don't need to tell you about taking medication for colds and flu: Because we all take it when we're not feeling well. You might have started taking other medication for other ailment, or started using diuretic drugs, to flush out excess water from your body.

There's millions of people who need to take antidepressants regularly such as: beta-blocker for some forms of migraine or heart problems.

The problem is: My research confirms that your panic attacks and related symptoms could have stemmed from any of the above, and these are just a few I've pulled out of the hat, there's plenty more rabbits in there.

The fact remains: Panic attack aren't pleasant by no means and the feelings in themselves, make you feel like there is something seriously wrong with you. This makes you worry even more.

Now this next very important decision is: One of the biggest mistakes we all make in these similar circumstances. We join the millions of other people who run to the doctors for some hopeful advice.

I'm sure you won't need three guesses to decipher what the scribbled writing on the prescription says? You nailed it in one! A course of antidepressants.

Don't get me wrong, these do help, for the short term period of four to five weeks. Well that is until: You have to be upgraded to a higher dosage, or you need to be weaned off. Either way the symptoms are going to come flooding back with a vengeance.

Luckily you have the great initiative to help yourself by reading this book. I would have gladly done the same, if it was available to me at the time. When I was crying out for someone to help me. When I was desperate for someone to at leased give me some idea, of what was happening to me.

I couldn't find any answers, because no one new anything about panic attacks. It took me nearly three years before I was lucky enough to root out the cause and cure myself.

Well at least by downloading this book you have taken a step in the right direction, and you are going to find out and understand exactly what is happening to you.

This will enable you to cure yourself completely from those strange and frightening feelings that: If not pinpointed and addressed could last the rest of your life.

In the next chapter you will find a short story of how I first experienced panic attack. You will probably be able to relate to some of the symptoms. But my main reason for including this story is in relation to your initial outcome.

Chapter 4
My Panic Attack Experience

I had always classed myself as being quite fit and very rarely visited the doctors, for any sort of ailment. I used to exercise pretty regularly with weights, and at the time I was holding down three jobs.

One of those jobs, was a contract Public Service Vehicle Driver, and on this particular morning the contract was to take some disabled children to school.

The weather was frosty and quite cold for a September morning, but I must admit, I felt absolutely great. I had just recently turned forty, and I felt stronger and fitter than I ever had.

The bus I was driving was all kitted out with a hydraulic lift, floor clamps and straps to accommodate wheel chairs.

My job this particular day, was to go and pick up a school escort from her home, and then drive to various other addresses picking children up for school.

When I was at my third address, I started feeling a bit out of breath. I had just loaded a wheel chair into the bus via the hydraulic lift, and while I was knelt down fastening the floor clamps to the bottom of the wheelchair, I started struggling to breathe, and I felt the floor clamps were getting harder to tighten.

Just then I noticed a few drops of water dropping on the floor next to my hand, while at the same time, realizing it wasn't the floor clamps that were getting harder, I was gradually getting weaker.

As I struggled to get up off the floor, I could feel sweat rolling down the side of my face, and then trickling down the back of my neck. I eventually made my way to the front of the bus and slid back into the driving seat.

By this time my breathing had got worse, so I tried desperately to not think about it, and concentrated on continuing on my journey. A few minutes later, I felt a strange sharp sensation on the left side of my neck, which was quickly followed by a tight feeling in my chest.

I stopped the bus at the side of the road, and mentioned to the school bus escort, who I was working with at the time, that I would have to go out and get some air.

She quickly replied that: I looked as white as a ghost, which didn't make me feel any better. Then suddenly I felt a strange tingling and numbness sensation proceeded to spread all over my body.

So I started to walk up the street to get to the back of the bus, and away from the widows, and out of sight of the children. Because I didn't want them to see how frightened I really was.

Every step I took my breathing got heavier, making it harder to walk. I lent my arms on the top of a dry stone wall, while I looked over into some fields. All I could see was bits of blurry green and brown Shapes, due to my vision being all hazy and out of focus.

I desperately tried to stop myself from thinking, "It's a heart attack, I'm going to die, so what happens now?" I started feeling a weird tingling sensations all over my body, followed by a low pitched humming sound deep inside my head.

I started really struggling to breathe, and the only thing I could think of to take my mind off all of this was: To keep telling myself to, "listen to the birds."

The school escort had already knocked on one of the house doors, and asked the woman occupier, if she could use her telephone to ring for an ambulance. The woman amazingly happened to be a nurse, who had already brought a blanket out, which she gently placed over my shoulders.

By this time I was gasping for air, hunched up with my head down, and walking around in fairy steps trying to keep myself alert.
The nurse put her arms around me and led me to the garden wall.

She then asking me to sit-down until the ambulance arrives, while positively reassured me: I wasn't going to die, as I had already asked her to tell my wife that I love her, and say goodbye to my three kids.

I was hooked up to a heart monitor, and supplied with an oxygen mask on the way to the hospital. While I was continually repeating to myself, "just five more minutes and I'll be safe." I tried to focus on the light on the ambulance roof, because everywhere I tried to look was making me feel dizzy and nausea.

The ambulance crew wheeled me into a room in the hospital, where the nurse hooked me up to another heart monitor. I was still shaking from head to foot an hour later, when my wife, Susan, came in to see me.

She looking relieved because, on her way in, she had just caught sight of the ambulance crew, looking at the tail end of the heart monitor readout, showing a flat line, so she greeted me with a kiss on the oxygen mask.

The doctors decided to keep me in for observation, and more tests to monitor my heart. Then two days later they came to the conclusion, that it must have been a panic attack, so I was allowed home.

After days of being at home, I was still trembling from head to foot, and finding it hard to concentrate on anything. My breathing was all wheezy, as if my lungs were all clogged up, and the day light hurt my eyes.

Adding to all the other symptoms, was a kind of distorted blurred vision. So I ended up going down to the doctors, where I came away with a prescription for a bottle of beta-blocker pills and a salbutamol asthma inhaler.

I must state: That the last time I had to take any sort of medication, for any type of ailment. Was after breaking my leg, 16 years previous. But this was completely different, pain I'm able to cope with, but strange uncanny feelings, like you were going to die is a different story all together.

The easiest way to describe a small part of these feelings is: They are similar to going down the steep end of the big dipper, and your stomach is churning. Or when some one grabs you from behind and makes you jump.

The feelings may only last two or three seconds normally, but to someone with a similar nervous condition to what you have and what I had, it could last hours, days or even weeks.

What makes it even worse is: you haven't the foggiest idea of what is happening to you, and apparently neither does anyone else. Panic attacks have been around since us humans have. so why on earth in the year 2018 are we only just finding out about them.

The fact is: If you are unfortunate enough to experience panic attacks, nobody seems to have a clue, you're just left in the cold trying to sort them out yourself. You don't get any reassurance from people you think would know.

I must admit: I got fed up of trying to find out, because all I got was just a blank stare, followed by, "what do you think it is," or, "put your head between your legs, it will make you breathe better," or, "make an appointment with the nurse and she'll try syringing your ears out," and then, " take this course of pills and come back and see me in a weeks time."

The problem is, trying to explain what exactly is wrong with you. As far as you're concerned you might be the only person in the world with all these different ailments.

Then, because you haven't been to the doctors for a few years, you find out that all the rules have changed. They only wants to know about one ailment at a time. This makes you feel like you've been letting them all mount up, and you have made an appointment to sort out the job lot.

How can you put into words that:

"I have this continuous annoying humming noise inside my head."

"The lights in the DIY store hurt my eyes so I've got to walk around wearing sunglasses."

"The patterns on the carpet keep moving and I can't see things at the side of me."

"I can't work at the computer or watch the T.V. without feeling dizzy and nausea."

"I can't seem to concentrate on anything and I'm always feeling weird sensations."

"Looking at small tiles and paving stones when I'm out walking makes me feel strange."

"My heart keeps racing and I find it hard to breathe."

"The telephone and doorbell make me jump."

"I'm frightened to go outside and I can't stop shaking."

"I get muscle cramps in my hands, feet and stomach."

"I get night sweats, I can't sleep and I'm running to the bathroom all the time."

"I feel nervous and irritable and I keep getting chest and stomach pains."

It's just taken you an hour to get to the doctors, you're sat in the waiting room for twenty minutes, with everyone looking at you because your shaking from head to foot and gasping for breath.

Then you've got to try and explain what your symptoms are to your doctor, who thinks you're wasting his time if it's more than one ailment, which most of the time are unexplainable anyway.

I had to try something and these beta-blocker pills were all I had. I eventually managed to swallow one and sat down on the edge of a chair with my head in my hands, hoping that a miracle would happen, and this magic pill will make all my problems disappear.

An hour later I decided to take a walk outside for some air, but it was like I was walking in slow motion, in some sort of dream like state trying desperately to wake up.

The slabs on the pathway were making me feel dizzy, so I tried not to look at them, which turned out to be an impossible task. I couldn't breath and the buzzing in the back of my head was unbearable, so I ended up doing a u-turn arriving back home.

As the night went on by breathing got even worse. I was still sat on the edge of the chair shaking, and everything I looked at seemed to be wiggling around going out of focus.

Even the living-room lights used to hurt my eyes, causing me to wear sunglasses most of the time. I decided to try the salbutamol inhaler I was prescribed by the doctor. I inhaled it, held my breath for a few seconds, and it was like magic I could breathe again.

Two days later I went back to the doctor and told him that my breathing seemed to be under control, but I was still shaking from head to foot and my concentration was all over the place.

Chapter 5
How Not to Put an End to Panic Attacks

The doctor replaced the beta-blockers with anti-depressants and told me that I will have to be upgraded to some stronger ones in a couple of month's time.

Leaving the doctors my wife Susan and I decided to go for a drink. I was a bit nervous, in case someone noticed me shaking, but then again it might just calm me down a bit.

After three pints of lager and a couple of games of pool, I felt my normal self again, it was like all my symptoms had just vanished.

When we got home I threw the anti-depressants in the bin, I wasn't keen on taking pills as I said earlier, and it made matters worse thinking, "I'll have to start taking stronger one's later on."

The next day I did still feel strange but not as bad. I had a quick blow on my inhaler, which I was using about five times a day, and then I decided to catch up with some of my office work for my Entertainment Business.

Just short of an hour later I could feel the symptoms coming back, I had to try to avoid looking at the computer screen, eventually having to turn it off as it was making me feel nausea and dizzy.

I just could not concentrate on what I was doing, my vision was blurred and the sunlight hurt my eyes. I had a constant humming in my ears, the back of my head and neck was all tight and aching and my heart felt like it was clawing its way out of my chest.

But what made matters even worse was: I couldn't even hold my pen to write as the trembling and muscle spasms decided to start. I eventually had to put my office work on hold, and ended up pacing up and down in the kitchen.

I finely retrieved a bottle of white wine out of the fridge, and ended up sitting down at the kitchen table. I poured myself a glass of wine, which I drank in a couple of quick mouthfuls.

For about ten minutes, my symptoms were twice as bad as they were originally. All I could do was prop my head up with my hands and wait for the wine to take effect, which it did on the second glass.

I had a gig that same night with the rock 'n' roll band I was singing with. I didn't really fancy slinging my self about on stage, but I didn't want to let the club or the rest of the guys down.

My wife Susan drove me to the venue, and set up most of the P. A. system. I had a couple of pints of lager and three glasses of white wine, and that helped me get through the night.

This same routine went on for over two years, were I was having panic attacks regularly and a lot of sleepless nights pacing around the living room floor.

I had got to the point were, I was frightened to leave the house or to answer the door, even the telephone used to make me jump out of my skin when it rang.

My brother in-law used to have to come and sit with me while my wife went out to work, because I was frightened of being left on my own.

My wife and kids had got fed up of not knowing what to do, when I used to cry and ask them for help. On top of that, I had gradually built my intake to a full bottle of wine per-day and six cans of Lager.

The feelings were getting more and more harder to control and I had reluctantly turned into an alcoholic. Yes, I was in a right state, I went from a six-foot, fifteen stone weightlifter, to a ten stone weakling.

Chapter 6
The Last Straw

Not only that: My mouth and tongue were constantly swollen, in harmony with my purple and chapped lips. I was vomiting all the time and everything else that went with it.

The last straw came, when I was singing Unchained Melody in a public house with the band. I started crying half way through the song and so were most of my friends in the audience, including my wife. They all knew if I didn't sort myself out within the next couple of months, I would probably be dead.

Early the next morning I woke up in bed, curled up, face down on my right side. This being the only position I could breathe in. My stomach ache alarm clock reminded me that I was still alive.

I made it to the bathroom for once without loosing any body fluids, until I could sit down with my chin in the sink. I remember looking in the bathroom mirror at a forty-two year old man in a well-aged skeleton body.

I eventually made it down the stairs and got sat on my living room chair, picking up the glass of wine where I had left it three hours before. I reluctantly tried to force the wine down my throat as it was like acid burning my mouth.

It took three hours and a full bottle of wine, before my body stopped shaking and all the other symptoms subsided, then an additional can of lager and the odd glass of wine every hour to keep the feelings at bay.

I decided to try and take one of the diazepam pills that I had acquired four days earlier, due to a spell in hospital. I though it was a bit risky after the amount of alcohol I had consumed but I was desperate.

I was in a world of my own and like a zombie for two hours, when the symptoms started coming back. I was determined not to have any more alcohol, so I decided to try and have a sleep on the couch.

I managed a couple of hours, before the feeling got the better of me and woke me up with a vengeance. I asked my wife Susan to ring the hospital, and find out how long I would have to wait before I could take another diazepam pill.

She came back with the reply, "not less than eight hours," so that was it, I was on my own for at leased four hours. I sat down in my normal position, on the edge of living-room chair.

I seemed to be fighting a loosing battle, with the muscle spasms in my hands and feet, and the constant nagging in my stomach.

I asked Susan to turn the television up, so I couldn't hear the unbearable buzzing in my head, and try to drown the noise of my chair vibrating from side to side.

The patterns on the carpet seemed to be wriggling worse than ever, but I was determined to give it my best shot. Susan stopped up with me all that night, as I must admit I was frightened of being left on my own.

I had already past my diazepam deadline, but I decided to try and last as long as I could without taking one, I knew they were there if worse came to worse.

I had gone twenty-four hours drug and alcohol free, replacing it with tonic-water, hoping the quinine will assist me in some way. I was still trembling and all the other symptoms were all present.

I remembered reading somewhere that: "Given half the chance your body has the power to heal itself." After all the things we've been through together, I was determined to give it every chance it needed.

Chapter 7
How I Put an End to Panic Attacks

I knew I had to take it one day at a time, repeating to myself in my mind, "I will feel a lot better tomorrow." After another sweating, trembling and sleepless night on the couch, I managed to glance through some books, a friend of mine had left for me.

The books were all about stress and anxiety, and although they helped me to take my mind of my ailments for a while, they didn't really appeal to me much, because most of the information was more about how the nervous system works.

I was cold and shaking all over, and going to bed was the only way I could think of to keep myself warm, and I knew before anything else, I would have to fight my alcohol problem first.

It took a good two weeks of constant trembling, and a lot of running to the bathroom, for the alcohol withdrawals to subside. Every day I
told myself that "I would feel better tomorrow," and I definitely did.

I knew I had to root out my nervous disorder, and to do that I decided the best way would be: To go back in time to before the panic attacks happened. Taking me back to the beginning of this story, September 1996.

Eight weeks before I had the panic attack on the bus, I received a letter from the doctors surgery, asking me to make an appointment for a check up, because I had not been to the doctors for the last three years.

So I ended up having to go to the doctors twice, because both times my blood pressure reading was up. This meant I had to go to the hospital to have my blood tested.

When the results came back the cholesterol levels were high, so the doctor put me on a six-week low fat diet. I was determined to get the levels down, because the doctor warned me that a possible heart attack could occur within the next two to ten years.

Obviously this made me a lot more conscious of my eating habits.

So I started on the diet for about two weeks, until the food started to get really boring. I thought missing the odd meal or two would help me loose weight quicker.

Then the odd meal or two turned into, hardly any food at all. Just before the six weeks of my diet was up, I had lost over two stone in weight. Oddly enough, that is when I experienced my first panic attack on the bus.

So it was obvious that this strict diet had caused the panic attack, in the first place. So at leased I had a place to start my study, and the first area had to be: **Cholesterol and cholesterol levels**.

This took me back to my first visit to the doctors, two days after coming out of hospital. While I was there trying to explain to the doctor about all my problems, he told me that my results from my blood test had come back from the analysts.

He went on to say: that my cholesterol level results, were absolutely brilliant. Not only that: Apparently one of the cholesterol levels was the lowest the doctor had ever seen.

I asked the doctor "what exactly are cholesterols?" "And with one being that Low, could this have had something to do with my problems?" He told me he didn't really know, and that all he knew was that they had to be low.

I decided to start more research on cholesterol and found out that: Cholesterol is a natural steroid made by the liver, from a variety of foods.

It is an important constituent of body cells, that are involved in the formation of hormones, and in the transport of fats in the bloodstream to tissue throughout the body, in the form of lipoproteins.

Lipoproteins are particles with a core made up of cholesterol and fats, in a varying proportion with an outer wrapping of phospholipids, which consists of cell membranes and nerve tissue.

The proportion of lipoproteins consists of three major classes, High Density, Low Density and Very Low Density. The High-Density lipoproteins (HDL) are what our bodies produce from food sources manufactured in our liver, which is sometimes called the janitor or the good cholesterol.

HDL goes around our blood stream, cleaning up the harmful effects left by the bad cholesterol. Good food sources of HDL can be found in: Blueberries, oranges, plant oils, various nuts, avocados, rice, bran, sunflower seeds, green peas and various oily fish.

The other two lipoproteins LDL and VLDL, are known as the bad cholesterol, found in: egg yolks, red meat, cheese, butter and saturated fats. which are absorbed into our bodies, via our digestive system, thought to be the main culprits for the furring of the arteries and various other problems.

So it's a good idea to balance these cholesterols. If you have more of the good cholesterol, (HDL) this counter acts the bad cholesterol (LDL) and (VLDL) cholesterols and visa versa.

When the doctor told me that: There was one cholesterol that he had never seen so low. It more than likely was, the good cholesterol HDL. This is probably why? I suddenly developed a breathing condition.

Because cholesterol is: a natural steroid, and one of It's many functions is: to moderate the opening and closing of the oxygen valves in the blood stream.

There's also a proven association between low cholesterol level, and the presence of major depression, in patients with panic disorders.

Don't forget: Your body can't produce these vital chemicals and must be obtained from the food you eat: Your diet directly affects the brain chemicals, that influence your emotional reactions. Such as: mood and behaviour, and you need two types of essential fatty acids from the food you eat to build healthy brain cells.

These two important components are: Alpha-linolenic acid, which is the foundation of the omega 3 family. Good food sources are: flax seeds, chia seeds, walnuts, sea weed, green leafy vegetables, and cold water fish like salmon, sardines, mackerel, and trout.

The second essential fatty acid you need is: Linoleic acid, this is the foundation of the "omega-6" family of fatty acids. Good food sources are: Vegetable oil, cold-pressed sunflower oil, safflower oil, corn oil, sesame oils, nuts, chicken, turkey and potatoes.

From these two acids your brain can make (docosahexaenoic acid) DHA and (arachidonic acid) AA, the longer chained fatty acids that are incorporated in it's cell membranes.

These more complex fatty acids are also available, preformed, directly from food.

This is very important in our case, because the brain's ability to assemble these fatty acids, can be compromised by stress, infections, alcohol, excess sugar, and vitamin or mineral deficiencies, all the factors common today.

Fatty acids are the key building blocks to a healthy brain and certain fatty acids have been shown to actually boost intelligence. So an imbalance of fatty acids are thought to be linked to hyperactivity, depression, brain allergies, and schizophrenia.

Healthy monounsaturated fats are also found in: avocados, peanuts, walnuts, almonds, pecans, chicken, beef, turkey, eggs, mackerel, and herrings, as well as in sesame, palm, corn, sunflower, and soybean oils.

Just like essential nutrients, amino acids, and essential fatty acids from the omega oils, the body requires saturated fat. Cell membranes are made up of both unsaturated and saturated fatty acids, which means the body needs a variety of fat sources.

Without these fat sources, cells lose their stiffness, and are unable to function properly. We should eat foods with saturated fat so our body can absorb and utilize other essentials, such as: fat soluble vitamins and minerals.

Essential fatty acids need the more stable saturated fats in order to remain in the body tissue and to contribute to a healthy immune system.

So as you can see: we are very close to finding out why we are having these panic attacks, and because I was not eating properly the obvious other category would be: **vitamin deficiency**.

Vitamins are a group of organic substances that are essential for the normal functioning of our bodies. As the body only manufactures two of these vitamins, niacin and vitamin D, it is essential that we obtain the other eleven vitamins from our food.

I was not interested in five of these vitamins A, D, E, K and B12 because these are stored in our liver for up to two years, and a daily intake is not necessary.

The vitamins I concentrated my research on: Were mainly in the vitamin B complex, such as: Pantothenic acid, riboflavin, thiamine and pyridoxine. These are all water-soluble vitamins, which our bodies cannot hold for very long, even if taken in excess.

These vitamins are regularly excreted in the urine, therefore a portioned intake of these vitamins, at least twice a day is essential, especially if you are on a poor diet.

Please note: if you come under any of the following categories you are susceptible to a deficiency in these vitamins, leading to a chemical imbalance. This undoubtedly could be adding to the cause of stress related symptoms such: as panic attacks.

Poor diet, drink alcohol regularly, take diuretic drugs, take antidepressant drugs, take blood pressure drugs, take antipsychotic drugs, take oral contraceptives, take corticosteroid drugs, take laxative drugs, excessive intake of coffee or extremely profuse sweating.

Pantothenic Acid is responsible for the manufacture of sex hormones and corticosteroid hormones. It is also responsible for the utilization of other vitamins, the functioning of the nervous system and the adrenal glands.

A deficiency usually occurs as a result of alcohol dependency, diuretic drugs (I'll tell you more about diuretic drugs later) or a strict or very poor diet.

The principle effects of a deficiency of pantothenic acid are muscle cramps, tingling and numbness sensations, respiratory problems, nausea, fatigue, and abdominal pains. Good food sources of this vitamin are: egg yolk, fish, liver, kidney, vegetables and wheat germ.

Thiamine or Vitamin B1: Plays a vital role in the activity of various substances, that promote a chemical reaction in the body, and in the functioning of the nerves, muscles and heart.

People susceptible to a B1 deficiency are those on a poor diet such as: white flour and sugar products, and people with an over active thyroid. A deficiency may cause: irritability, loss of appetite, sleeping problems, depression, memory loss and abdominal pain. Good food sources of this vitamin are: bran, pasta, pork, liver, whole meal bread, fish, nuts, eggs and beans.

Riboflavin or Vitamin B2 is essential for: the breakdown of carbohydrates, proteins and fats, and is responsible for the production of energy in cells and hormones via the adrenal glands.

A deficiency of riboflavin such as: a poor diet, alcohol dependency and diuretic drugs, can cause certain temporary vision or eye disorders. Where as: the subject is abnormally sensitive to sun light
or bright lights, and finds it hard to read and focus on objects.

Other B2 deficiency disorders are: chapped lips and soreness of the tongue and mouth. Good food sources of this vitamin are: eggs, milk, cheese and whole grain.

Pyridoxine or Vitamin B6 is: involved in the break down of proteins, carbohydrates and fats, and also the manufacture of red blood cells and antibodies.

Pyridoxine is also involved in the functioning of the digestive system, nervous system and in the maintenance of healthy skin. People susceptible to B6 deficiency are those on a poor diet, people treated with certain drugs and people with alcohol problems.

B6 deficiency causes depression, irritability, swollen mouth and tongue, weakness, trembling, skin disorders, cracked lips and sometimes seizures. Good food sources of this vitamin are: pork, liver, chicken, beans, potatoes, and bananas.

Diuretic drugs are more commonly known as water tablets: Because they are used to increase urine production. Their main use is to remove fluid from tissue, by reducing the amount of water in the circulation.

Diuretic drugs are normally given to patients to relieve fluid retention that causes ankles to swell, bloating and breast tenderness. They are also used to lower blood pressure and for this reason they are sometimes given to patients with Meniere's disease (a disorder of the inner ear).

The unfortunate people with Meniere's disease are: constantly experiencing panic attacks, and stress related illnesses. Although these have nothing what so ever to do with the disease itself.

The problems these people are experiencing, like many on prolonged use of diuretic drugs, are due to: These drugs cause an increase urine production. This washing all the water-soluble B vitamins out of their system.

Not only is all the above vitamin deficiency true, but also adding to their problem is: A deficiency of potassium in the blood, with adverse effects such as: dizziness, drowsiness and muscle weakness.

There's also a deficiency in magnesium with an adverse effect such as: anxiety, restlessness, tremors, palpitations, and depression.

Natural Diuretics: When your body doesn't get enough B vitamins it tends to accumulate excess fluids. This leads to water retention around the lower legs and abdomen, leading to bloating.

The doctor then gives you diuretic drugs to combat this: Which starts the vicious cycle all over again. If you have water retention there is such a thing as: Natural diuretics that increases the flow of urine, and aids in the removal of fluids from the body.

This also means the loss of B vitamins and minerals that you will have to replenish regularly. Good food sources of these natural diuretics are: raw onions, tomatoes, lettuce, carrots, cabbage, Brussels sprouts, beets, asparagus, cranberry juice, apple cider vinegar, fennel seeds or plant, oats, radish, celery, parsley, artichokes, water cress, melons, juniper berries, nettles, dandelions, yarrow, linden, coffee, tea and coke.

The fact is: all these symptoms related to the one's I was having, the similarities were too great to be anything else. All the doctor had to say to me: "More than likely your body is short of B vitamins."

All I really needed was a diet sheet containing vitamin B sources, and a bit of information on how vitamins work, and that would have been the answer to most of my problems.

It would have saved my family and me years of unnecessary stress. That's what this book is all about: Routing out and analysing the causes of your problems. Looking back and pinpointing the possible causes and correcting them, before they have a chance to get any worse.

I started my recovery by: Eating products, which were full of B vitamins on a daily basis, such as: marmite on toast, liver, beans, eggs, mackerel, whole wheat cheese sandwiches, and nuts.

I could actually feel the symptoms disappearing one by one, as if someone had just pulled an invisible blanket off from over my head. I just kept on telling myself " I'll feel even better tomorrow," and every day I did feel better.

Sometimes: usually at night, the feelings would try to come back. So all I used to do was: Get up and make myself a drink of tea, and eat some mackerel in tomato sauce on toast or in a sandwich, then the feelings just used to disappear.

I read somewhere that: Your brain can only think of one thing at a time. So while I was recovering I started changing my way of thinking, by finding something to occupy my mind, most of the feelings would just last a couple of minutes, and then disappear.

I still was quite a bad sleeper: I used to jump maybe fifteen times per night, as if something kept on startling me just before I was about to dream.

I must admit those days I was quite a bad sleeper and on the odd occasion I used to jump slightly but nowhere near as bad. I found that if I emptied my mind and thought of nothing at all, I could gradually get back to sleep.

I used to change my way of thinking by quickly changing my thoughts to different topics. If I started to experience anything that resembled a panic attack, I quickly picked a book or magazine up and started to read anything that was written down.

I knew these feeling were just an imprint in my mind of the experiences I use to have, so I was determined not to let them get the better of me.

I even moved a piano into the living room and learned how to play it. I started doing some DIY around the house. Then one day when I had overdone a weightlifting session, I was really out of breath and I very nearly thought to myself "I can't breath," but I quickly picked my guitar up which was the nearest thing at hand, and started singing anything that was in my head at the time.

I didn't give the feelings a chance to surface and they never did. Just put these feelings out of your mind completely and they will never return, unless you go back to your old ways.

I found that experimenting with different foods worked as well, such as garlic, red chilly powder, mustard, raw onions, beetroot, marmalade, chocolate, and bananas etc, which all have various calming properties triggering natural body chemicals to your aid.

For instance when you chew something hot like curry or a raw onion, or even a sip of hot coffee. Your brain automatically thinks your mouth is on fire, and quickly releases calming chemicals all over your body, which work instantly.

Garlic has got that many healing properties you wouldn't believe: Anti-cancer, lowers blood pressure, lowers cholesterol, antibacterial, antiseptic, anti-mucus, and anti-microbial properties.

Recent studies have shown that: garlic reduces the hardening of the arteries that mostly appears with age. Garlic is also used to stimulate the production of white blood cells and is regarded by many health practitioners as a first line treatment for infectious diseases.

I use garlic instead of antibiotics, for instance just recently I had a massive abscess on the roof of my mouth which I tried using various mouthwashes to no avail. I ended up chopping up two clothes of garlic and mixed them with a bit of brown sauce on the side of my plate, I then used it to dip my snack in.

I got up the next morning and the abscess had completely gone and it hasn't been back since. There is a lot of natural foods that really do work, honey, ginger etc, you might have to experiment a bit to find the right one for you, but that's what it's all about.

Some foods used to make me feel ill when I was using alcohol as a sedative these included things containing chocolate or coffee. The obvious reason of course was that these are stimulants, which are counteracting the sedative, in other words, sobering you up.

The other trick I have found to work well is singing. Try singing to yourself out loud. Not only does it take your mind off any problems that might be bothering you, singing is the best exercise you could wish for to get your breathing back into it's normal rhythm, and is also an excellent exercise for your diaphragm.

I must admit I never liked to sing at home at all, I was a bit embarrassed about it, now, my wife can't shut me up, and I've heard her singing to herself in the kitchen a few times as well.

Our bodies know how to breathe all by themselves, the problem is when we intervene we seem to get it wrong. Diaphragm breathing is using the lower part of your body, if your shoulders are moving when you inhale, you are breathing wrong.

Chapter 8
Conclusion

Which brings me up to the present day September 2018. I haven't had a panic attack for the last 20 years. The last time I went to the doctors was for a medical to renew my PCV license. And that was a year ago. I have felt absolutely great.

All the symptoms have been gone now for that length of time, apart from the odd wheeze or two here and there. I can seriously say at 62 years old I feel even better than I did before my incident.

I speak to people quite regularly who have been using alcohol and antidepressants for over eight years or more, for similar kinds of problems to what I was having.

They tell me how they would love to be able to either stop drinking or not have to take medication to function, and nine times out of ten these people are on a very poor B vitamin diet.

Not only that these same people are taking diazepam and also drinking alcohol as well, which is going to make their problems ten times worse. I was also surprised to find out: How many millions of young people are being prescribed anti-depressants regularly, with no questions asked or any attempt to route out the cause of their problems.

Where as in most cases especially the girls who are watching their figure, tend to eat a minimum of the wrong types of food anyway. A well-documented survey over the last fifty years, has been uncovered just recently claiming that people have and still are being diagnosed with having stress or anxiety to suit which ever anti-depressant is out on the market at the time of diagnosis.

Drug manufactures have been paying millions to doctors to promote these drugs, and some of the anti-depressants with minimal or no side affects, have only just come to light, as being the main causes of violence in the household.

It is the most natural thing in the world to have some sort of stress, we were born with it, every one of us needs a certain about of it to survive in every thing we do 24 hours a day, everyday of our lives.

We used stress originally to help us get out of sticky situations when an animal wanted us for their main course, in the days when we were dragging our partners around by the hair and bashing each other with clubs.

These days it is used to stop you getting run over by a truck or preparing you for protection against any kind of threat. It can kick in at lightening speed anytime, anyplace, anywhere.

When it does kick in, it quickly raises your heartbeat to provide blood to your muscles, just in case you are going to have to jump or run or fight.

For the extra blood your heart has just acquired from all the different areas of your body that has been temporarily shut down, you are going to need more oxygen, that's why you start to breath heavier.

In unison with your heart, lungs and muscles, all of your five senses, sight, sound smell, touch and taste have just been boosted up to super power ready to help you fight your attacker.

The problem is: if you haven't nourished there special abilities with the correct vital vitamins they don't work correctly and that is where your problems evolve.

You could be just sat watching T. V. when the strange feelings start and make you feel ill. You start to get all tensed up sat there dwelling and worrying about why your hearts started racing ten to the dozen.

All sorts of thoughts are going through you head at this point, you may be thinking you are having a heart attack or you're going to faint, this makes you worry even more.

Your start to make your heart beat faster. causing it to want more oxygen from your blood. This causes you to want to take in more oxygen, because you feel as if you can't breathe. (hyperventilation) So the more oxygen you try to take in, you find the harder it is to breathe.

This eventually will cause you to shallow breathe, (your bodies natural defence mechanism making you take short gasps or air) because your levels of carbon dioxide and oxygen have been disrupted, causing less oxygen to get through to your cells and vital organs, making you feel unable to get a good satisfying breath.

The longer this situation lasts, the more chance you have of experiencing a panic attack. Your subconscious mind has to get these oxygen and carbon dioxide levels back to normal. So if the shallow breathing does not work, then the only other alternative is to try and make you faint.

This would allow your body to adjust it's own breathing without you interfering, so you end up fighting a loosing battle against yourself. You see the problem is: your subconscious mind does not know the difference between fiction and reality.

So you only have to think about any sort of a threat, or start to worry too much about something that has not, and probably will never happen. Then all the above symptoms will automatically kick in to play, and constantly persist until you convince your subconscious that these thoughts have not actually happened.

The easiest way to stop these symptoms from occurring when they are not needed is to use the thinking exercises I talked about earlier, pick up a book and start reading anything out loud or sing a song to yourself.

If you're in the middle of town, obviously you don't really want to be singing at the top of your voice, so whistling a nice cheerful tune will soon get your oxygen level back to normal.

The natural way your subconscious deals with these situations is: to use the adrenalin up by way of: your emotions, such as: screaming or crying out loud like a baby does automatically. This actually kills two birds with one stone, by frightening your opponent away and bringing you aid.

Most people lose their stress by exercising, laughing, crying, shouting, screaming, singing, working and more or less just keeping active.

But if you only use a minimum of these actions, which is understandable if you: Have a lot on your mind for a relevantly long period of time, or you have a vitamin B deficiency, preventing the normal functioning of your body, and the manufacture of vital hormones.

The adrenalin level starts to build up and overflows into the bloodstream, whether you need it or not. One of the first signs you will notice instantly, usually when you are not involved in any physical exertion, is: Your heart starts to beat faster as it starts to receive an unexpected flow of extra blood, due to the adrenalin's chemical effect on the blood vessels, narrowing them to a minimum.

The second sign you will notice, is: How easy your breathing has become almost effortless, as the adrenalin causes the widening of your airways, in the preparation for the unknown. Ready to instantly oxygenate your blood at any slight inclination of stress.

These next symptoms are all simultaneously, caused by excess adrenalin. These are not necessarily in order, but they will all ring a certain bell inside your subconscious mind as soon as you read them. (As soon as I realized what was happening to me I was no longer afraid.)

As I said earlier, all of our five senses become super active. Your vision becomes too sensitive, causing bright lights to hurt your eyes, finding it difficult to read and focus on close up objects.

This is due to the adrenalin's effect on your eyes, which have now been transformed to pick up on any movement or minute detail or threat, directing your eyes forwards in a tunnel like vision.

You start hearing humming or annoying sounds in your ears or head, which are generally the sounds of the blood flowing through the veins in your eardrums.

You will find that your nose has become an excellent breathing tool, but you keep picking up on some annoying perfumes or smells that you have never noticed before.

Your hands and toes tingle as your touch becomes extra sensitive.

You start getting a strange metallic taste in your mouth, as your lips and tongue become extra sensitive.

Your stomach is aching or churning due to the adrenalin narrowing the blood vessels in the intestines.

You are getting tingling sensations all over your body, due to the adrenalin narrowing the blood vessels in your skin.

You are starting getting muscle cramps and stiffness, due to the extra blood flow and oxygenation of your muscles.

You feel the need to use the toilet often and are thirsty a lot of the time. This is caused by the corticosteroids, which are made by the adrenal glands, with one of their many functions being the control and excretion of water and salt in the urine, and will also be disposing of water soluble B vitamins, that will need to be replaced.

You often get throbbing headaches, which again adrenalin is one of the main causes. (I actually thought I was going mad at one point as I constantly tried to ease the pain by rubbing the back of my head.)

But as there are no sensory nerves in the brain, the narrowing of the blood vessels and the muscles tightening around the scalp and the back of the neck, combined with slight dehydration in the skin usually causes these headaches.

When we breathe in, the air in the lungs is diffused through cells and capillary walls into the blood plasma. The oxygen molecules combine with haemoglobin in the red blood cells to form oxyhemoglobin.

Once the blood reaches the body cells, carbon dioxide, which is now converted into carbolic acid, allows the oxygen to be released. This is why we need a balanced level of both carbon dioxide and oxygen to maintain a steady function of the body.

Your body needs a precise level of both gasses to reach its vital tissues and organs and once this balance is upset your body will do its utmost to get the balance back to normal.

I have tried to arm you with some sort of idea of the probable causes of the feelings you might be having at the moment and just to reassure you that: they are completely natural.

It is your body's way of rectifying the chemicals and at the same time telling you to do something about it. At leased you now know that you are definitely not on your own or in any kind of danger.

By trying these formulas I used, you will start to benefit within the next thirty minutes or so, and go on getting better each day until you are completely cured.

You must also understand that many doctors have never witnessed a panic attack, and unless they themselves have been a sufferer there can be little understanding of the problems and the overwhelming fear it produces.

By no means, is it the doctors fault: they are just doing their job to the best of their ability, by treating the symptom rather than the cause.

They rely on the fact that: many ailments are corrected by the bodies own immune system. But I really think that the health system needs to come out of the stone age, and stop thinking we all need electric shock treatment, when their methods don't and never will work.

Just for instance: If you went to the hospital now with chest pains and unable to breathe, they would suspect you were experiencing a heart attack, and automatically give you pure oxygen. When in fact: You are hyperventilating and oxygen would definitely be the worse thing they could give you.

This is why we are drawn to look elsewhere, to try and get some sense out of the people who have experienced, the same sort of feelings that we are encountering, and be able to cure ourselves without being used as a guinea pig in the process.

The doctors are not experienced in anxiety, and panic attack disorders. So after you have suffered for a few months with him trying out his new batches of drugs on you, that haven't worked, he then refers you to a psychiatrist for another few months of behaviour therapy and deep breathing exercises.

Fair enough these exercises would calm anyone down who "wasn't" suffering from panic attacks. But as soon as you do experience one, these breathing exercises involving taking deep breaths actually make you worse.

I know when I was struggling and fighting to breathe, all the nicest, calming and soothing words didn't mean a thing to me, and the last thing on my mind was to sit back and relax and take nice deep breaths, who are they kidding.

How can you sit back when your stomach muscles are all contacting into cramps, as well as your legs and arms. When your trying you hardest to find the best position to help you to breathe better in.

When you are frightened and thinking you are about to die, worrying about what is going to happen to you and how will your family cope.

This is why I say: They haven't a clue what we experience, and until they do, they are fighting a loosing battle at our expense. Your body gets it right first time and we need to listen to who knows best.

When your body starts to shallow breath try to cope with it as long as you can. When I was sat alone trying to think about different subjects, I found that: If I stood up and tried to walk around the room pretending to talk to someone on the telephone helped.

Then of course there is the singing exercises I talked about earlier which defiantly will work for you. Once you start to get your diet back to normal I can seriously say, all this will be a thing of the past and you will forget about it completely.

Unless of course like me you choose to help other people and relive all your experiences over, and over again. The only difference being is: knowing what we know now: they can't hurt us anymore.

We all have a certain amount of ailments, aches and pains due to everyday wear and tear. If we sat down and dwelled on them for long enough, we can actually make them worse by just thinking about them.

The idea is to put these out of your mind completely, and keep telling yourself: "You feel absolutely great." Do this every morning when you wake up and every-time you feel a little low.

You are what you think you are, and you have the power to alter your thoughts in to good ones. Make your thoughts work for you not against you. We all go through a learning experience in everything we do, most of which is trial and error.

I firmly believe the main culprit for stress related symptoms such as panic attacks, is: essential fats and vitamin B deficiency. One of the main effects of any sort of stress is loss of appetite, and one of the side affects to the drugs I mentioned earlier, including regular alcohol consumption is: dehydration and loss of appetite.

It is estimated that a third of the population are already taking antidepressants for stress related illnesses. This is great for the drug companies but not so great for the patient. Because there has to come the time when these so called masks will fail to work.

The more you resort to using modern day medical treatments, the more you will come to depend on them, the symptoms are merely suppressed with the cause still remaining.

I'm not saying it's easy, it's the hardest thing I have ever done in my life, but its well worth it. All you have to do it cut down; don't take the easy way out.

In a strange sort of way I am glad it happened to me, because not only has it made me see things in a different light, as it certainly has enlightened me, and given me some idea of what other people are going through right at this very moment.

But it has definitely made me start and go for every goal, that I have only really thought about. And the great news is: Once your chemicals are back to normal, it's almost impossible to revert back. As long as you keep feeding the furnace.

This book is a true account of what happened to me. It's intensions are to help others, who are suffering from stress related symptoms. By shedding some light on, a delicate subject not talked about enough.

Please read this book over a few more times, to get the best result.

The information will cure you like it has me, and I know once you start and get your body chemicals back to normal, you will be better than you were before the panic attacks.

P.S. Don't forget: keep me posted on your outcome.
aleccmoir@gmail.com
                         Kind regards,
                                    Alec C Moir.